Transformed: A Comprehensive Guide to Modern Gender-Affirming Surgeries

by Megan Dennis

"Discover a comprehensive and empowering guide that explores the diverse options and considerations surrounding transgender surgery, providing valuable insights, support, and information for individuals seeking to navigate their personal journey of gender affirmation.

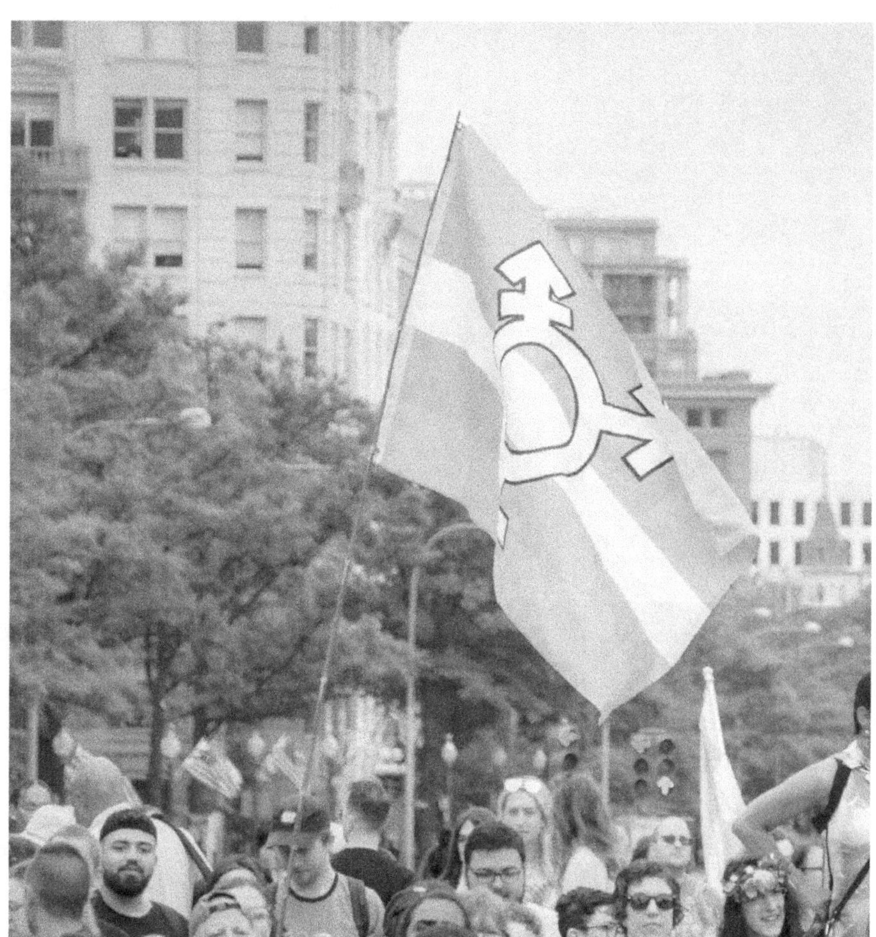

Contents

1

Introduction

1. Defining gender identity and exploring the spectrum of gender diversity.

Welcome to the exciting journey of exploring gender identity and the beautiful spectrum of gender diversity! In this chapter, we'll dive into the fascinating world of gender, discussing what it means to embrace and express our true selves.

Imagine a colorful tapestry where gender isn't limited to just "male" and "female." Instead, it encompasses a vast and diverse range of identities. Gender identity is how we personally experience and understand ourselves in terms of being male, female, a combination of both, or neither. It's an inherent and deeply personal aspect of who we are.

Now, let's address a common misconception: gender identity is not determined by our physical appearance or the sex assigned to us at birth. While many people's gender identity aligns with their assigned sex, others may experience a disconnect, giving rise to the concept of being transgender. Transgender individuals have a gender identity that differs from the sex they were assigned at birth.

The beautiful thing about gender is that it exists on a spectrum. It's not simply a binary choice between male and female, but rather a rich tapestry of identities. Some individuals may identify as genderqueer, non-binary, genderfluid, or agender, just to name a few. Each person's gender journey is unique and valid, deserving of respect and understanding.

By exploring the spectrum of gender diversity, we can celebrate the full range of human experiences and challenge societal norms that limit our understanding of gender. It's about embracing the freedom to be ourselves, to express our gender in a way that aligns with our true identity.

In the following chapters, we'll delve deeper into the experiences and challenges faced by transgender individuals, the role of gender-affirming surgeries, and the incredible possibilities that lie ahead on the path of self-discovery and self-acceptance.

So, let's embark on this journey together, with open hearts and open minds, as we celebrate the kaleidoscope of gender identities that make our world so wonderfully diverse.

References:

1. **American Psychological Association. (2020).** Answers to Your Questions About Transgender People, Gender Identity, and Gender Expression. Retrieved from https://www.apa.org/topics/lgbt/transgender.pdf

2. **National Center for Transgender Equality. (n.d.).** Understanding Non-Binary People: How to Be Respectful and Supportive. Retrieved from https://transequality.org/issues/resources/understanding-non-binary-people-how-to-be-respectful-and-supportive

3. **Human Rights Campaign Foundation. (n.d.).** Glossary of Terms. Retrieved from https://www.hrc.org/resources/glossary-of-terms

4. **GLAAD. (n.d.).** Transgender FAQ. Retrieved from https://www.glaad.org/transgender/faq

2. **Embracing the Journey:** Navigating the Transition Process with Confidence

Congratulations! You've taken the exciting step of exploring your gender identity and embracing your true self. The journey of transitioning can be an incredible adventure of self-discovery, but we understand that it can also feel overwhelming at times. Fear not! In this section, we'll provide you with guidance and support as you navigate the transition process.

First and foremost, remember that transitioning is a deeply personal journey. There's no one-size-fits-all approach, and the path you choose is entirely up to you. Take the time to reflect on your desires, aspirations, and goals for your transition. Seeking guidance from mental health professionals and support networks can be immensely helpful as you embark on this transformative journey.

One essential aspect of the transition process is developing a solid support system. Surrounding yourself with understanding and accepting individuals—friends, family, or members of the LGBTQ+ community—can provide the emotional support you need. Support groups and online communities can also offer a safe space to connect with others who share similar experiences.

As you navigate the transition process, it's crucial to consider various factors, including legal and financial considerations. Understanding the legal aspects related to changing your name, gender marker, and accessing healthcare can help you plan your transition effectively. Additionally, exploring insurance coverage and financial resources available for gender-affirming procedures can alleviate some of the financial burdens associated with transitioning.

While it's essential to have patience and compassion for yourself through-out the journey, it's equally important to educate yourself about the available resources and options. Understanding the different avenues of transition, including social, medical, and legal aspects, empowers you to make informed decisions about your path forward. From hormone therapy to gender-affirming surgeries, each step requires careful consideration and consultation with knowledgeable healthcare professionals.

Remember, transitioning is not a linear process. It's a series of steps and experiences that are unique to each individual. Some individuals may choose to socially transition first, experimenting with changes in pronouns, clothing, or appearance, while others may opt for medical interventions like hormone therapy or gender-affirming surgeries. There's no right or wrong way to transition—it's all about what feels right for you.

By embracing the journey, you're taking an active role in shaping your authentic self. Embrace the freedom to explore, experiment, and express your gender identity in ways that feel most genuine to you. Your journey is valid, and you deserve to be seen, respected, and celebrated for who you are.

References:

5. **National Center for Transgender Equality. (n.d.).** Name and Gender Change 101. Retrieved from https://transequality.org/documents/name-and-gender-change-101

6. **World Professional Association for Transgender Health. (2011).** Standards of Care for the Health of Transsexual, Transgender, and Gender-Nonconforming People. Retrieved from https://www.wpath.org/media/cms/Documents/SOC%20v7/SOC%20V7_English.pdf

7. **Human Rights Campaign Foundation. (n.d.).** Transgender Health and Wellness. Retrieved from https://www.hrc.org/resources/transgender-health-and-wellness

8. **National LGBTQIA+ Health Education Center. (2016).** Clinical Guidelines for Transgender Primary Care. Retrieved from https://www.lgbtqiahealtheducation.org/wp-content/uploads/Clinical-Guidelines-for-Transgender-Primary-Care_2ndEdition_2016.pdf

3. **Exploring Resources:** Navigating Legal and Financial Considerations with Confidence

Transitioning is an exciting and empowering journey, but we understand that it can come with its fair share of logistical considerations. Fear not, intrepid explorer! In this section, we'll guide you through the maze of legal and financial aspects of transitioning, helping you navigate them with confidence.

Let's start with the legal side of things. As you embark on your transition, you may consider changing your name and gender marker to reflect your true identity. This process varies by jurisdiction, so it's important to familiarize yourself with the specific requirements and procedures in your area. Seeking legal counsel or utilizing online resources can help you navigate the name and gender change process smoothly and securely.

Additionally, understanding your legal rights and protections is crucial. Familiarize yourself with the laws and policies in your jurisdiction that protect individuals from discrimination based on gender identity. Knowing your rights empowers you to advocate for yourself and ensures that you're treated fairly and respectfully in various areas of life, such as employment, housing, healthcare, and public accommodations.

Now, let's dive into the financial considerations of transitioning. Gender-affirming procedures, such as hormone therapy and surgeries, can be expensive. However, don't be discouraged—there are resources available to help alleviate the financial burden. Start by exploring your health insurance coverage. Many insurance plans now recognize the importance of gender-affirming care and may cover certain procedures. Review your policy carefully, paying attention to exclusions and coverage criteria.

If your insurance does not provide adequate coverage, or if you don't have insurance, there are organizations and programs that offer financial assistance for gender-affirming surgeries. Research local and national funding options, grants, and scholarships specifically designed to support transgender individuals in their journey. Community-based organizations and LGBTQ+ advocacy groups often have information and resources available.

Crowdfunding platforms can also be a valuable tool to raise funds for gender-affirming surgeries. With the support of friends, family, and allies, you can share your story and rally community support to help cover the costs. Online communities and social media can provide a platform to amplify your campaign and connect with individuals who are passionate about supporting transgender individuals.

Remember, financial considerations should not deter you from pursuing your true identity. While the path may present challenges, there are avenues of support and resources available to help you overcome financial barriers. By actively seeking out these resources, you can navigate the financial aspects of transitioning with confidence and focus on your personal growth and well-being.

So, fear not the legal and financial aspects of your journey, dear explorer. Armed with knowledge, resources, and a supportive community, you can navigate these considerations with confidence, ensuring that nothing stands in the way of your authentic self.

References:

9. **National Center for Transgender Equality. (n.d.).** ID Documents Center. Retrieved from https://transequality.org/documents/id-documents-center

10. **Human Rights Campaign Foundation. (n.d.).** Know Your Rights: Employment. Retrieved from https://www.hrc.org/resources/know-your-rights-employment

11. **National Center for Transgender Equality. (n.d.).** Know Your Rights: Housing. Retrieved from

https://transequality.org/issues/housing

12. **Lambda Legal. (n.d.).** Transgender Rights. Retrieved from https://www.lambdalegal.org/issues/transgender-rights

2

Exploring Gender-Affirming Surgeries

1. The Power of Choice: Understanding Gender-Affirming Surgeries

Ahoy, fellow adventurer! Welcome to the realm of gender-affirming surgeries—a place where individuals can shape their bodies to better align with their true selves. In this section, we'll embark on a journey to explore the transformative power of these surgeries and the diverse options available to individuals seeking gender affirmation.

Gender-affirming surgeries, also known as transgender surgeries, are medical procedures designed to help align one's physical characteristics with their gender identity. These surgeries can be life-changing, empowering individuals to feel more comfortable and authentic in their bodies. It's important to note that not all transgender individuals pursue surgical interventions, as each person's journey is unique and personal. The decision to undergo gender-affirming surgery is a deeply personal choice that should be made in consultation with healthcare professionals and based on individual needs and goals.

Now, let's set sail and explore the sea of options when it comes to gender-affirming surgeries. The available procedures encompass various aspects of the body, allowing individuals to customize their transition based on their desired outcomes. Here are some of the common types of gender-affirming surgeries:

1. **Chest (Top) Surgeries:** For transgender men (assigned female at birth) and non-binary individuals seeking a flatter chest, chest masculinization surgeries can help achieve a more masculine appearance. These procedures, such as bilateral mastectomy or breast reduction, involve removing excess breast tissue and reshaping the chest contour.^[17]

2. **Genital (Bottom) Surgeries:** Genital reconstruction surgeries, also known as gender confirmation surgeries or "bottom surgeries," are performed for transgender individuals seeking to align their genitalia with their gender identity. These procedures are highly individualized and can involve various techniques, including vaginoplasty (creation of a vagina), phalloplasty (creation of a penis), or metoidioplasty (enhancement of the clitoris for transgender men).^[18]^[19]

3. **Facial Surgeries:** Facial feminization surgery (FFS) and facial masculinization surgery (FMS) can help individuals modify facial features to align with their gender identity. FFS may include procedures such as forehead contouring, rhinoplasty (nose reshaping), and jawline feminization, while FMS may involve procedures like jawline augmentation and chin reshaping.^[20]^[21]

4. **Voice Surgeries:** Some individuals may choose to undergo voice feminization surgery (VFS) or voice masculinization surgery (VMS) to modify their voice pitch and resonance to better match their gender identity. These procedures involve techniques to alter the vocal cords and vocal tract.^[22]

It's essential to note that these surgeries, like any medical procedures, come with potential risks and considerations. Consulting with experienced healthcare professionals, such as plastic surgeons and urologists specialized in transgender care, is crucial to understand the specific procedures, potential outcomes, and associated risks.

Remember, dear explorer, the power of choice rests in your hands. The journey of gender affirmation offers a treasure trove of surgical options to help you sculpt your body to better align with your true self. Stay curious, stay informed, and most importantly, stay true to your authentic identity as we continue this adventure together.

References:

13. **American Society of Plastic Surgeons. (n.d.).** Gender Confirmation Surgery. Retrieved from https://www.plasticsurgery.org/reconstructive-procedures/gender-confirmation-surgery

14. **World Professional Association for Transgender Health. (2021).** WPATH Clarification on Medical Necessity of Treatment, Sex Reassignment, and Insurance Coverage for Transgender and Gender-Diverse Individuals. Retrieved from https://www.wpath.org/media/cms/Documents/Web%20Transfer/Resources/171204%20WPATH%20Clarification%20on%20Medical%20Necessity%20of%20Treatment%20Full%20Packet.pdf

15. **Crane, C. N., & Oates, J. F. (2006).** Reconstruction of the Neophallus. In E. J. Sanfilippo (Ed.), Operative Obstetrics and Gynecology (2nd ed., pp. 1491-1505). Taylor & Francis.

16. **Morrison, S. D., & Crane, C. N. (2018).** Gender Confirmation Surgery. In A. Thaller (Ed.), Plastic Surgery (pp. 1419-1438). Springer.

17. **Bluebond-Langner, R., & Berli, J. (2021).** Chest Wall Masculinization and Contouring. In S. E. Santucci & A. J. Jordan (Eds.), Gender-Affirming Surgery: Principles and Techniques (pp. 315-324). Thieme.

18. **Chen, M. L., & Schechter, L. S. (2020).** Vaginoplasty. In J. L. Caplan & S. J. Hricak (Eds.), Taylor and Francis' Atlas of Gender Affirmation Surgery (pp. 33-48). CRC Press.

19. **Crane, C. N. (2020).** Phalloplasty. In J. L. Caplan & S. J. Hricak (Eds.), Taylor and Francis' Atlas of Gender Affirmation Surgery (pp. 49-74). CRC Press.

20. **Facialteam. (n.d.).** Facial Feminization Surgery (FFS). Retrieved from https://facialteam.eu/facial-feminization-surgery-ffs/

21. **Keojampa, B. K. (2018).** Facial Feminization Surgery. In A. Thaller (Ed.), Plastic Surgery (pp. 1651-1666). Springer.

22. **Department of Otolaryngology-Head and Neck Surgery, University of California, San Francisco. (n.d.).** Voice and Communication Therapy for Clients Who Are Transgender/Transsexual. Retrieved from https://transcare.ucsf.edu/guidelines/voice

2. **Navigating the Seas of Preparation:** Preoperative Considerations and Care

Ahoy, brave explorer! As you set sail on the path of gender-affirming surgeries, it's essential to navigate the seas of preparation with care and attention. In this section, we'll equip you with the knowledge and understanding to embark on your surgical journey with confidence and preparedness.

Preparing for gender-affirming surgery involves a series of important considerations and steps to ensure a successful and smooth experience. While each surgery and individual is unique, here are some general preoperative considerations to keep in mind:

1. **Finding the Right Surgeon:** The journey begins with finding a skilled and experienced surgeon who specializes in gender-affirming surgeries. Seek recommendations from healthcare professionals, local LGBTQ+ organizations, and online communities. Schedule consultations with potential surgeons to discuss your goals, ask questions, and assess their approach and expertise in transgender care.

2. **Mental and Physical Health Evaluation:** Prior to surgery, healthcare professionals will conduct thorough evaluations to assess your mental and physical health. These evaluations may include discussions about your gender dysphoria, medical history, and any preexisting conditions that might impact surgery or recovery. Mental health support is vital throughout the process, and working closely with mental health professionals can ensure you're prepared emotionally and psychologically.

3. **Hormone Therapy:** For individuals undergoing genital reconstruction surgery, hormone therapy may be a significant factor in the preparation process. Depending on your desired outcomes, hormone therapy can help facilitate the development of secondary sex characteristics that

align with your gender identity. Your healthcare provider will guide you on the appropriate timing and management of hormone therapy in relation to surgery.

4. **Preoperative Assessments and Tests:** Your surgical team will perform various preoperative assessments and tests to ensure your safety and well-being. These may include blood tests, electrocardiograms (ECGs), and imaging studies. These assessments help identify any underlying conditions and determine your eligibility for surgery.

5. **Lifestyle Adjustments:** As you prepare for surgery, making certain lifestyle adjustments can contribute to optimal outcomes and recovery. These adjustments may include quitting smoking, maintaining a healthy diet, engaging in regular exercise, and following any specific preoperative instructions provided by your surgical team.

Remember, dear explorer, that preparation is key to a successful voyage. Collaborate closely with your surgical team, adhere to their guidance, and communicate openly about your expectations and concerns. By navigating these preoperative considerations with diligence and care, you're setting yourself up for a transformative and fulfilling surgical experience.

Now, steady your course as we sail forth into the next chapter, where we'll dive deeper into the intricacies of the surgical procedures themselves. Anchors aweigh!

References:

23. **World Professional Association for Transgender Health. (2021).** Standards of Care for the Health of Transsexual, Transgender, and Gender-Nonconforming People. Retrieved from https://www.wpath.org/media/cms/Documents/SOC%20v7/SOC%20V7_English.pdf

24. **American Society of Plastic Surgeons. (n.d.).** Gender Confirmation Surgery: What to Expect. Retrieved from https://www.plasticsurgery.org/reconstructive-procedures/gender-confirmation-surgery/what-to-expect

25. **Daskalakis, D. C., & Mayer, K. H. (2017).** Surgical Care for Transgender and Gender Nonconforming Individuals. In Fenway Guide to Lesbian, Gay, Bisexual, and Transgender Health

(2nd ed., pp. 440-446). American College of Physicians.

26. **Bluebond-Langner, R., & Berli, J. (2018).**

27. **American Society of Plastic Surgeons. (n.d.).** Gender Confirmation Surgery. Retrieved from https://www.plasticsurgery.org/reconstructive-procedures/gender-confirmation-surgery

28. **Djordjevic, M. L., Stojanovic, B., Bizic, M., & Kojovic, V. (2018).** Metoidioplasty: Techniques and outcomes. Translational Andrology and Urology, 7(4), 723-731. doi: 10.21037/tau.2018.06.13

29. **Sutcliffe, P. A., Dixon, S., Akehurst, R. L., Wilkinson, A., Shippam, A., White, S., ... Richards, C. (2009).** Evaluation of surgical procedures for sex reassignment: A systematic review. Journal of Plastic, Reconstructive & Aesthetic Surgery, 62(3), 294-306. doi: 10.1016/j.bjps.2007.11.018

3. Navigating the Surgeon's Toolkit: Understanding Surgical Procedures and Techniques

Ahoy, intrepid adventurer! Welcome to the heart of the surgical voyage. In this section, we'll dive deep into the surgeon's toolkit, exploring the various gender-affirming surgical procedures and techniques available to shape your body according to your true identity. So, buckle up—our destination is a world of transformation and possibility.

1. **Chest (Top) Surgeries:** For those seeking to embark on a chest-transforming journey, top surgeries offer a spectrum of possibilities. If you're a transgender man or non-binary individual seeking a flatter chest, bilateral mastectomy or breast reduction can help sculpt a more masculine appearance[31]. For transfeminine individuals, breast augmentation is an option to enhance and feminize the chest area. The surgeon's skillful hands and artistic vision, guided by your desires, will help shape a chest that embodies your authentic self.

2. **Genital (Bottom) Surgeries:** Ah, the realm of bottom surgeries— the sea of transformation where individuals can align their genitalia with their true selves. Vaginoplasty, the creation of a neovagina for transgender women, involves skillful surgical techniques to construct a functional and aesthetically pleasing genital structure[32]. Phalloplasty, on the other hand, sets sail on a different course, navigating the creation of a neophallus for transgender men. This intricate procedure often involves multiple stages and can utilize techniques such as flap phalloplasty or metoidioplasty with urethral lengthening[33]. Remember, each journey is unique, and the specifics of these surgeries will depend on individual needs and goals.

3. **Facial Sculpting:** In the realm of facial transformation, facial feminization surgery (FFS) and facial masculinization surgery (FMS) shine as beacons of possibility. FFS encompasses a range of procedures, from brow contouring and rhinoplasty to jawline feminization and lip augmentation[34]. On the flip side, FMS offers techniques like jawline

augmentation and chin reshaping to help forge a more masculine facial structure. The surgeon, armed with expertise and an understanding of your desired outcomes, will navigate the contours of your face to unveil the truest version of yourself.

4. **Voice Harmonization:** The quest for a voice that resonates with your authentic self can take you on a journey of voice harmonization surgeries. Voice feminization surgery (VFS) aims to raise the pitch and modify the resonance of the voice for transgender women, while voice masculinization surgery (VMS) adjusts the pitch for transgender men. Skilled surgeons work their magic, employing techniques to refine the vocal cords and shape the sound that emanates from within^[35]. With their expertise, you can embark on a voyage of vocal transformation, finding a voice that aligns with your identity.

As you navigate the surgeon's toolkit, remember that each procedure requires careful consideration and collaboration with your healthcare team. Expertise, experience, and understanding are the compass points that guide your surgical journey. So, set your sights on the horizon, embracing the transformative power of these surgical techniques, as we sail forth into a world where authenticity and self-expression reign.

References:

30. **World Professional Association for Transgender Health. (2021).** Standards of Care for the Health of Transsexual, Transgender, and Gender-Nonconforming People. Retrieved from https://www.wpath.org/media/cms/Documents/SOC%20v7/SOC%20V7_English.pdf

31. **American Society of Plastic Surgeons. (n.d.).** Gender Confirmation Surgery. Retrieved from https://www.plasticsurgery.org/reconstructive-procedures/gender-confirmation-surgery

32. **Djordjevic, M. L., Stojanovic, B., Bizic, M., & Kojovic, V. (2018).** Metoidioplasty: Techniques and outcomes. Translational Andrology and Urology, 7(4), 723-731. doi: 10.21037/tau.2018.06.13

33. **Sutcliffe, P. A., Dixon, S., Akehurst, R. L., Wilkinson, A., Shippam, A., White, S., ... Richards, C. (2009).** Evaluation of surgical procedures for sex reassignment: A systematic review. Journal of Plastic, Reconstructive & Aesthetic Surgery, 62(3), 294-306. doi: 10.1016/j.bjps.2007.11.018

Charting the Course: Preparing for Gender-Affirming Surgery

1. The Voyage Begins: Preparing Mind, Body, and Soul for Surgery

Ahoy, courageous voyager! As you embark on the exhilarating journey towards gender-affirming surgery, it's essential to prepare your mind, body, and soul for the adventure that lies ahead. In this section, we'll set sail into the depths of preparation, equipping you with the tools and knowledge to navigate this transformative voyage with grace and confidence.

1. **Mental and Emotional Preparation:** Your inner compass is as crucial as the surgical compass in guiding your journey. Take time to nurture your mental and emotional well-being before surgery. Seek support from therapists, support groups, or online communities that specialize in transgender care. Engage in self-care practices, such as mindfulness, journaling, or artistic expression, to cultivate resilience and emotional balance. Remember, dear sailor, taking care of your mental health is paramount on this transformative expedition.

2. **Establishing a Support Network:** A crew of support can help navigate the challenging waters of surgery and recovery. Reach out to friends, family members, or chosen family who are affirming and understanding. Educate them about the surgical process, so they can provide the love, support, and assistance you may need along the way. Building a strong support network ensures you have anchors to rely on when the tides get rough.

3. **Preparing Physically:** As you prepare your vessel (your body) for the

voyage, it's important to follow any preoperative instructions provided by your surgical team. These may include adjustments to medications, dietary guidelines, or restrictions on certain activities. Engaging in regular exercise and maintaining a balanced diet can help optimize your physical health, ensuring a smoother journey. Remember to consult with your healthcare provider to develop a personalized plan that fits your unique needs and circumstances.

4. **Surgical Consultation and Planning:** Ahoy, captain! The next step is to schedule a consultation with your surgeon. During this voyage of collaboration, discuss your goals, desires, and any concerns you may have. Your surgeon will navigate the seas of information, providing detailed explanations of the surgical procedure, potential risks, and expected outcomes. Together, you'll chart a course that aligns with your aspirations, ensuring a shared understanding and mutual trust.

5. **Financial Considerations:** Navigating the financial aspect of surgery is an important part of the journey. Insurance coverage, if available, can significantly impact the affordability of gender-affirming surgeries. Explore your insurance policy's provisions related to transgender healthcare and discuss coverage options with your healthcare provider and insurance company. Additionally, investigate financial assistance programs and resources that can provide support in funding your surgical expedition.

As you prepare for this monumental voyage, remember that your journey is unique to you. Embrace the excitement, the uncertainties, and the empowerment that lie ahead. By taking care of your mind, body, and soul, and building a supportive network around you, you'll be ready to set sail towards the destination of authenticity and self-discovery.

Fair winds and smooth seas, brave explorer, as we venture forth into the next chapter, where we'll explore the intricacies of the surgical experience itself.

References:

34. **[36] World Professional Association for Transgender Health. (2021).** Standards of Care for the Health of Transsexual, Transgender, and Gender-Nonconforming People. Retrieved from https://www.wpath.org/media/cms/Documents/SOC%20v7/SOC%20V7_English.pdf

35. **The Trevor Project. (n.d.).** Support for Transgender and Nonbinary Youth. Retrieved from https://www.thetrevorproject.org/trvr_support_center/transgender

36. **Bockting, W., Coleman, E., Deutsch, M. B., Guillamon, A., Meyer, I., Meyer, W. J., ... & Samons, S. L. (2016).** Adult development and quality of life of transgender and gender nonconforming people. Current Opinion in Endocrinology, Diabetes and Obesity, 23(2), 188-197. doi: 10.1097/MED.0000000000000226

37. **Saraswat, A., Weinand, J. D., & Safer, J. D. (2015).** Evidence supporting the biologic nature of gender identity. Endocrine Practice, 21(2), 199-204. doi: 10.4158/EP14351.RA

2. Riding the Waves: Navigating the Surgical Experience and Recovery

Ahoy, intrepid adventurer! You've reached a critical juncture in your journey—the surgical experience itself. As you prepare to ride the waves of transformation, it's important to familiarize yourself with what to expect during and after gender-affirming surgery. In this section, we'll be your trusty navigators, guiding you through the surgical voyage with a mix of playfulness and seriousness.

1. **Setting Sail:** The Big Day: Picture this—it's the morning of your surgery, and the excitement is palpable. You'll check in at the hospital or surgical center, where the friendly crew of medical professionals will prepare you for the voyage ahead. They'll explain the steps, answer any last-minute questions, and make sure you're comfortable before you set sail into the operating room.

2. **Anesthesia:** As you embark on this deep sea adventure, the anesthesiologist will administer anesthesia, guiding you into a state of gentle slumber. They'll keep a watchful eye on you throughout the surgery, ensuring your safety and comfort as the surgeon sets to work.

3. **The Surgeon's Expertise:** Like skilled mariners, surgeons navigate the intricate waters of your body with precision and care. They'll employ advanced techniques and modern tools to bring your desired changes to life. Whether it's reshaping your chest, sculpting your face, or refining your genitalia, their expertise will be the compass that guides your transformation.

4. **Time at Sea:** The duration of your surgery will depend on the specific procedure and your unique circumstances. It may feel like time has slowed as the surgical team skillfully works towards your goals. But fear not, dear adventurer, for every minute spent at sea brings you closer to the shores of your authentic self.

5. **Emergence from Slumber:** As the surgery concludes, you'll gradually awaken from your slumber, finding yourself in the recovery room. The caring crew of nurses and doctors will be there to monitor your progress, ensuring your comfort and well-being. Though you may initially feel groggy, rest assured that you're on your way to a smoother recovery.

6. **Navigating the Postoperative Seas:** Recovery from surgery is like navigating uncharted waters. You'll receive detailed instructions from your surgical team on wound care, medications, and follow-up appointments. It's important to adhere to these guidelines diligently, as they will contribute to a successful and comfortable recovery.

7. **Support Along the Way:** As you sail through the postoperative seas, a support network becomes even more crucial. Reach out to your loved ones, friends, and healthcare providers for guidance and assistance. They'll be your life rafts, helping you navigate any challenges that arise, and celebrating every milestone achieved on your journey to wholeness.

8. **Weathering the Emotional Storms:** Remember, dear voyager, that the surgical journey can bring forth a range of emotions. It's natural to experience a mix of excitement, relief, and occasional moments of uncertainty. Be kind to yourself, practice self-compassion, and seek support when needed. The storm clouds will pass, revealing clear skies and a newfound sense of authenticity.

As you navigate the surgical experience and recovery, keep your eyes fixed on the horizon of your true self. Ride the waves with resilience, trust in your surgical team, and lean on the support of those who love and understand you. Soon, you'll stand tall on the shores of your dreams, ready to embrace the boundless possibilities that await.

3. Treasure Chest: Self-Care and Emotional Well-being during Recovery

Ahoy, resilient voyager! As you navigate the waters of recovery after gender-affirming surgery, it's essential to tend to the treasure chest that is your self-care and emotional well-being. This chapter will be your compass, guiding you through the playful and serious aspects of this crucial phase.

1. **Rest and Recharge:** Your body has embarked on a remarkable transformation, and now it needs time to heal. Rest and relaxation become the wind in your sails during recovery. Settle into a cozy nook with your favorite books, movies, or music, and let your mind and body rejuvenate. Remember, dear adventurer, that recovery is not a race but a voyage that requires patience and self-compassion.

2. **Wound Care:** Ahoy, matey! Caring for your surgical wounds is a vital part of the recovery journey. Follow the instructions provided by your surgical team to keep your wounds clean and protected. Gently navigate the seas of wound care, using the prescribed ointments or dressings. If any concerns or questions arise, don't hesitate to reach out to your healthcare provider for guidance.

3. **Nourishing the Body:** A balanced diet becomes your trusty first mate during recovery. Focus on nourishing your body with nutrient-rich foods that promote healing and vitality. Ah, but don't forget to indulge in a few treats along the way—a piece of dark chocolate or a slice of your favorite pie can be the windfall that lifts your spirits.

4. **Gentle Movement:** While rest is crucial, gentle movement keeps the ship of your body sailing smoothly. Engage in light activities approved by your healthcare provider to promote circulation and prevent stiffness. Take short walks along the beach, practice gentle stretching, or indulge in peaceful yoga sessions. Let your body guide you, finding the balance between rest and movement.

5. **Emotional Whirlpools:** The recovery journey can stir up a whirlpool of emotions. It's natural to experience a range of feelings, from elation and gratitude to moments of vulnerability or frustration. Give yourself permission to navigate these emotional waters with self-compassion. Seek solace in journaling, talking to supportive friends or professionals, or engaging in creative outlets that allow your emotions to find expression.

6. **Seeking Support:** Ahoy, fellow adventurers! Remember that you're not alone on this voyage. Reach out to your support network, including friends, family, or support groups, to share your experiences and seek guidance. They can provide a listening ear, words of encouragement, and a sense of belonging during moments of uncertainty or celebration.

7. **Celebrating Milestones:** As you sail through recovery, be sure to celebrate the milestones achieved along the way. Each step forward, no matter how small, is a triumph worth acknowledging. Celebrate with joy and gratitude, whether it's removing bandages, resuming activities you love, or feeling more at home in your transformed body. Cheers to the victories, and remember that you are the captain of this ship.

Dear voyager, as you navigate the seas of recovery, tend to the treasure chest within you—self-care and emotional well-being. With rest, nourishment, movement, and support, you'll sail through this phase with resilience and grace. The treasures you discover along the way will be the resilience, strength, and self-discovery that empower you to embrace the vast horizon of your authentic self.

References:

38. [44] World Professional Association for Transgender Health. (2021). Standards of Care for the Health of Transsexual, Transgender, and Gender-Nonconforming

Navigating the New Horizons: Life After Gender-Affirming Surgery

1. Anchors Aweigh: Embracing Your Authentic Self and Building Confidence

Ahoy, intrepid explorer! You've reached the shores of your authentic self, transformed by the voyage of gender-affirming surgery. As you step into the uncharted waters of life after surgery, it's time to embrace your new-found identity and build the confidence to navigate this brave new world. In this section, we'll be your trusted navigators, guiding you through the playful and serious aspects of this exciting chapter.

1. **Embracing Your Authentic Self:** Congratulations on reaching this milestone, brave adventurer! As you embark on life after surgery, take a moment to reflect on the profound journey you've undertaken. Embrace your authentic self with love, compassion, and acceptance. Let go of any lingering doubts or societal expectations, and anchor yourself in the truth of who you are. Remember, dear explorer, your identity is valid, and you have the power to shape your own narrative.

2. **Building Confidence:** Like a sturdy ship, confidence is your anchor as you navigate the tides of life. Building confidence post-surgery is a gradual process that involves self-reflection, self-care, and self-expression. Take the time to celebrate your achievements, both big and small. Surround yourself with positive influences, supportive communities, and role models who inspire you. As you become more comfortable in your skin, your confidence will grow, allowing you to set sail towards your dreams.

3. **Exploring Self-Expression:** Life after surgery opens up a world of possibilities for self-expression. Whether it's through fashion, hairstyles, or personal style, embrace the freedom to express yourself authentically. Play with colors, patterns, and textures that resonate with your truest self. Consider exploring hobbies and activities that bring you joy and allow you to express your unique interests and talents. Remember, dear adventurer, self-expression is a compass that guides you towards a fulfilling and authentic life.

4. **Navigating Relationships:** As you navigate your post-surgical journey, relationships may evolve or change. Some connections may deepen and flourish, while others may require adjustments or even departures. Surround yourself with individuals who affirm and respect your true identity, creating a support network that understands and celebrates your journey. Open communication, empathy, and understanding will be your guiding lights as you navigate the interpersonal seas.

5. **Advocating for Yourself and Others:** Your journey has equipped you with a wealth of knowledge and experience. Use your voice and newfound confidence to advocate for yourself and others in the transgender and gender-nonconforming community. Participate in advocacy organizations, raise awareness about transgender issues, and promote inclusive policies and practices. Together, we can create a more accepting and affirming world for all.

6. **Continued Growth and Learning:** Life after surgery is a continual voyage of growth and learning. Stay curious, embrace new experiences, and seek opportunities for personal and professional development. Engage in ongoing self-reflection, reassessing your goals and aspirations along the way. Remember, dear voyager, that growth comes from embracing the unknown and embracing the infinite possibilities that lie ahead.

As you set sail into the vast ocean of life after gender-affirming surgery, trust in your inner compass, embrace your authentic self, and let the winds of confidence carry you forward. The journey may have had its challenges, but the rewards of self-discovery, resilience, and empowerment await you on this new horizon.

2. Mapping the Seas: Nurturing Well-being and Resilience

Ahoy, resilient voyager! As you chart the course of life after gender-affirming surgery, it's important to navigate the seas of well-being and resilience. In this section, we'll be your trusty cartographers, guiding you through the playful and serious aspects of nurturing your overall well-being.

1. **Self-Care:** Ah, the art of self-care—a treasure worth cherishing! Take time each day to engage in activities that nourish your body, mind, and soul. It could be as simple as savoring a cup of tea, practicing mindfulness or meditation, indulging in a bubble bath, or venturing into the great outdoors. Self-care is like a lighthouse, guiding you through the storms and helping you maintain balance and harmony in your life.

2. **Prioritizing Physical Health:** Your body is a magnificent vessel that deserves to be cared for. Prioritize your physical health by adopting healthy habits such as regular exercise, nutritious eating, and sufficient sleep. Consult with healthcare professionals for routine check-ups and screenings. Remember, dear adventurer, that your body is your ally on this journey, and taking care of it allows you to fully embrace the adventures that lie ahead.

3. **Mental and Emotional Well-being:** Nurturing your mental and emotional well-being is like having a sturdy anchor amidst the waves. Seek support from therapists, counselors, or support groups who specialize in gender-affirming care. Explore techniques such as journaling, creative expression, or talking openly with trusted friends or loved ones. Remember, dear voyager, it's okay to ask for help when you need it—the bravest explorers often rely on the support of others.

4. **Building Resilience:** Life is a sea of constant change, and resilience becomes your compass in navigating the waves. Cultivate resilience by embracing challenges as opportunities for growth, reframing setbacks as learning experiences, and practicing self-compassion. Surround yourself

with positive influences and engage in activities that strengthen your resilience, such as pursuing hobbies, engaging in meaningful work, or connecting with a supportive community.

5. **Finding Purpose and Meaning:** A life well-lived is anchored in purpose and meaning. Explore activities, causes, or careers that align with your values and bring a sense of fulfillment. Volunteer for organizations that champion transgender rights, share your story to inspire others, or embark on a path of self-discovery through education or creative pursuits. By navigating the waters of purpose, you can create ripples of positive change in both your life and the world around you.

6. **Celebrating Milestones:** Life after surgery is filled with milestones worth celebrating. Each achievement, no matter how small, represents a step forward in your personal journey. Whether it's landing a job, completing an educational program, or advocating for transgender rights, take the time to acknowledge and celebrate your accomplishments. Surround yourself with friends and loved ones who can raise a toast to your resilience and achievements.

7. **Embracing Joy and Gratitude:** Ah, the sweet nectar of joy and gratitude! Savor the moments of happiness that come your way, no matter how fleeting. Embrace gratitude for the resilience, support, and opportunities that have guided you on your path. Capture these moments by creating a gratitude journal or expressing your appreciation to those who have supported you. In the sea of life, joy and gratitude become your guiding stars, illuminating the way forward.

Dear voyager, as you navigate the seas of well-being and resilience, remember to honor and nurture yourself. From self-care to resilience-building, and from finding purpose

3. Setting Sail: Nurturing Relationships and Building Support Networks

Ahoy, social navigator! As you set sail into the vast ocean of life after gender-affirming surgery, it's time to nurture relationships and build a strong support network. In this section, we'll be your friendly crewmates, guiding you through the playful and serious aspects of fostering meaningful connections.

1. **Anchoring Authenticity:** Authenticity becomes your guiding star as you navigate the waters of relationships. Be true to yourself and embrace your identity with pride. Share your story with those you trust, allowing them to see the depths of your journey. Remember, dear adventurer, that the people who appreciate and accept you for who you are will become the steadfast anchors in your life.

2. **Communication Compass:** Effective communication is the compass that helps you navigate the sometimes choppy waters of relationships. Practice open and honest communication, expressing your thoughts, feelings, and needs clearly and respectfully. Seek to understand others' perspectives and listen actively. Remember, dear voyager, that clear communication can help navigate misunderstandings and strengthen the bonds you forge.

3. **Chosen Family:** Family is not solely defined by blood but by the connections that anchor your heart. Build a chosen family of supportive friends, mentors, and allies who uplift and cherish you. These chosen family members will become your rock in times of need, providing love, acceptance, and understanding. Embrace the beauty of diverse relationships, knowing that family is not limited by traditional definitions.

4. **Allies and Advocates:** As you navigate the seas of life, allies and advocates become your invaluable crewmates. Seek out individuals who champion transgender rights and are committed to creating inclusive

spaces. Engage with organizations, both local and global, that promote equality and advocate for transgender rights. Together, you can sail towards a more accepting and affirming society.

5. **Building Boundaries:** Like setting sail with a sturdy ship, boundaries create a safe and respectful space in your relationships. Define your boundaries and communicate them clearly to others. Respect the boundaries of those around you as well. Boundaries allow for healthy relationships, where your needs are honored, and you can flourish as your authentic self.

6. **Sharing Experiences:** Your unique journey holds the power to inspire and educate others. Consider sharing your experiences through storytelling, writing, public speaking, or engaging in support groups. Your courage in sharing can provide hope and guidance to fellow voyagers on similar paths. Together, we can create a tapestry of shared experiences that fosters understanding and acceptance.

7. **Cultivating Empathy and Compassion:** In the vast ocean of relationships, empathy and compassion become your guiding stars. Seek to understand the experiences of others, showing empathy and compassion in your interactions. Support your fellow voyagers, lifting them up when they face challenges and celebrating their victories. By cultivating empathy and compassion, you create a nurturing environment where everyone can thrive.

As you navigate the seas of relationships and support networks, remember that you are not alone on this voyage. Surround yourself with anchors who uplift and embrace you. Together, we can create a community that celebrates diversity, fosters understanding, and sails towards a more inclusive world.

References:

39. [56] **National LGBTQ Task Force. (2021).** Creating Change: Tips for Being an Ally. Retrieved from https://www.thetaskforce.org/

40. **Human Rights Campaign. (2022).** Transgender Visibility Guide. Retrieved from https://www.hrc.org/resources/transgender-visibility-guide

41. **PFLAG. (2023).** Our Story. Retrieved from https://pflag.org/about

5

Beyond the Horizon: Sustaining Happiness and Fulfillment

1. The Joy of Discovery: Unleashing Your Passions and Pursuing Dreams

Ahoy, intrepid dreamer! Life after gender-affirming surgery is a vast canvas waiting to be painted with your passions and dreams. In this section, we'll be your enthusiastic cheerleaders, guiding you through the playful and serious aspects of sustaining happiness and fulfillment.

1. **Embracing Your Passions:** Ah, passions—the sparks that ignite your soul! Take the time to explore and embrace your interests, hobbies, and creative outlets. Engage in activities that bring you joy and fulfillment. Whether it's painting, writing, dancing, or tinkering with technology, allow your passions to be the wind in your sails. Remember, dear adventurer, that pursuing your passions is not only a source of happiness but also a way to express your authentic self.

2. **Setting Sail towards Dreams:** Dreams are like stars in the night sky, guiding you towards new horizons. Set sail towards your dreams, no matter how big or small they may seem. Identify your goals, break them down into actionable steps, and chart your course accordingly. Embrace the challenges and setbacks along the way, knowing that they are part of the grand adventure of pursuing your dreams.

3. **Creating a Vision Board:** Imagine having a visual map of your dreams and aspirations—a vision board! Gather images, words, and symbols that represent your goals and dreams. Arrange them on a board or a digital collage, creating a visual reminder of what you're striving for. Display

your vision board in a place where you can see it daily, allowing it to inspire and motivate you on your journey.

4. **Cultivating a Growth Mindset:** Like a mighty oak tree, a growth mindset allows you to bend and adapt in the face of challenges. Embrace the belief that your abilities and intelligence can be developed through effort, practice, and learning from setbacks. View challenges as opportunities for growth and approach them with resilience and curiosity. With a growth mindset, you can weather any storm and continue to evolve as a person.

5. **Balancing Work and Life:** As you sail towards happiness and fulfillment, it's important to find a balance between work and personal life. Prioritize self-care, leisure, and quality time with loved ones. Set boundaries around your work and honor your need for rest and rejuvenation. Remember, dear voyager, that a harmonious work-life balance allows you to thrive in all aspects of your life.

6. **Building Supportive Communities:** The journey towards sustained happiness and fulfillment is never meant to be taken alone. Surround yourself with supportive communities that share your values and interests. Seek out organizations, online forums, or social groups that align with your passions. Engage in meaningful connections and collaborate with like-minded individuals who inspire and uplift you.

7. **Paying It Forward:** As you experience the joy of sustained happiness and fulfillment, consider paying it forward. Support others on their journeys by sharing your knowledge, offering encouragement, or becoming a mentor. Engage in acts of kindness and contribute to causes that align with your values. By spreading joy and positivity, you create a ripple effect that touches the lives of others.

Dear dreamer, as you unleash your passions and pursue your dreams, remember that happiness and fulfillment are not distant shores but the very waves upon which you sail. Embrace the joy of discovery, chart your own course, and let the winds of passion carry you towards a life beyond the horizon.

References:

42. **Csikszentmihalyi, M. (1990).** Flow: The Psychology of Optimal Experience. Harper Perennial.

2. **Anchoring Well-being:** Cultivating Mindfulness and Gratitude

Ahoy, mindful explorer! As you navigate the seas of sustained happiness and fulfillment, it's time to anchor your well-being through the practices of mindfulness and gratitude. In this section, we'll be your cheerful guides, blending playfulness and seriousness to help you cultivate a joyful and grateful mindset.

1. **Embracing Mindfulness:** Picture this—a tranquil sea, clear skies, and the gentle rhythm of the waves. Mindfulness is your compass to navigate this serene state of being. Take a moment each day to tune into the present moment, embracing it fully without judgment. Engage your senses—feel the warmth of the sun, listen to the sounds around you, and savor the flavors of each experience. Mindfulness allows you to anchor yourself in the richness of the here and now.

2. **Mindful Breathing:** Your breath is like a faithful companion, always by your side. Take a deep breath, feeling the air fill your lungs, and release it slowly. Pay attention to the sensations of each breath, allowing it to ground you in the present. Whenever you feel overwhelmed or disconnected, return to the rhythm of your breath. It is your anchor amidst the ebb and flow of life.

3. **Gratitude Practice:** Ah, the power of gratitude—a treasure chest overflowing with joy! Take time each day to cultivate gratitude by acknowledging the blessings in your life. Reflect on the people, experiences, and opportunities that bring you happiness and fulfillment. Write them down in a gratitude journal, expressing your appreciation for each gift. Gratitude opens your heart to the abundance that surrounds you.

4. **Acts of Kindness:** Like a ripple in the water, acts of kindness spread joy and create a positive impact. Engage in small acts of kindness towards yourself and others. Extend a helping hand, offer a listening ear, or

perform random acts of kindness. Celebrate the interconnectedness of humanity and the power of compassion. With each act, you become a beacon of light in the lives of others.

5. **Cultivating Positive Mindset:** Your thoughts are like the wind, shaping the direction of your journey. Cultivate a positive mindset by intentionally shifting your focus towards the good in your life. Challenge negative thoughts and replace them with affirming and empowering ones. Surround yourself with positive influences, whether through uplifting books, inspiring podcasts, or supportive friendships. Remember, dear voyager, that a positive mindset propels you towards greater happiness and fulfillment.

6. **Self-Reflection:** The lighthouse of self-reflection illuminates the path to self-discovery. Set aside quiet moments to reflect on your experiences, emotions, and aspirations. Journal your thoughts, allowing them to flow freely onto the pages. Explore your dreams, desires, and fears with gentle curiosity. Self-reflection deepens your understanding of yourself, guiding you towards a life aligned with your truest desires.

7. **Mindful Relationships:** In the vast ocean of relationships, mindfulness creates a sacred connection. Engage in mindful listening, offering your full presence to others. Seek to understand their perspectives and experiences without judgment. Nourish your relationships by expressing gratitude, compassion, and love. With mindful relationships, you create a web of connection that brings joy and fulfillment.

As you anchor your well-being through mindfulness and gratitude, may your journey be filled with peace, joy, and a deep sense of fulfillment. Embrace the power of the present moment and let gratitude be the wind that carries you towards a life beyond your wildest dreams.

3. Nurturing Well-being: The Power of Connection and Purpose

Ahoy, fellow adventurer! As we continue our quest for sustained happiness and fulfillment, it's time to embrace the transformative power of connection and purpose. In this section, we'll be your enthusiastic guides, blending a playful spirit with the gravity of these profound concepts.

1. **Cultivating Meaningful Connections:** Imagine a treasure map leading you to a chest filled with priceless gems—the gems of human connection. Seek out meaningful relationships that enrich your life and bring you joy. Nurture friendships that resonate with your soul, surround yourself with people who lift you higher, and engage in heartfelt conversations that make your spirit soar. Remember, dear explorer, that the richness of life lies in the bonds we form with others.

2. **Authenticity and Vulnerability:** Peel back the layers of pretense and embrace your authentic self—the compass that guides you towards genuine connections. Show up as you are, with all your imperfections and vulnerabilities. Embrace the power of vulnerability, for it is the bridge that connects hearts and deepens relationships. Share your dreams, fears, and triumphs with those you trust, and allow them to do the same. In vulnerability, you'll find strength and acceptance.

3. **Community Engagement:** Picture a vibrant marketplace bustling with life—a community that thrives on connection and collaboration. Engage with your local community or join groups centered around your interests and passions. Volunteer your time, lend a helping hand, or contribute your unique skills to make a positive impact. Remember, dear changemaker, that by actively participating in your community, you become a catalyst for positive change.

4. **Finding Purpose:** Ah, purpose—the guiding star that illuminates your path and infuses your journey with meaning. Reflect on your passions, values, and the impact you wish to make in the world. Discover the

activities that ignite your soul, where time seems to stand still. Align your actions with your purpose, whether through your career, hobbies, or philanthropic endeavors. Embrace the knowledge that you are part of something greater than yourself.

5. **Growth and Learning:** Life is an ever-evolving adventure, and growth is the wind that propels us forward. Cultivate a growth mindset—a playful curiosity that embraces challenges, celebrates failures as stepping stones, and seeks opportunities for learning and self-improvement. Engage in lifelong learning, whether through books, courses, or exploring new fields of interest. Remember, dear learner, that growth is a lifelong voyage.

6. **Gratitude for Connection and Purpose:** Ah, the sweet nectar of gratitude—a potion that amplifies the power of connection and purpose. Take a moment each day to express gratitude for the meaningful relationships in your life and the purpose that drives you. Let gratitude fill your sails, propelling you towards deeper connections and a more purposeful existence. Celebrate the magic of gratitude and its ability to transform your perspective.

As you nurture your well-being through the power of connection and purpose, may your journey be filled with authentic relationships, meaningful experiences, and a sense of belonging. Embrace the profound impact you can have on others and the world, for together we can create a tapestry of joy, compassion, and purpose.

References:

43. [68] **Baumeister, R. F., & Leary, M. R. (1995).** The need to belong: Desire for interpersonal attachments as a fundamental human motivation. Psychological Bulletin, 117(3), 497–529.

44. [69] **Brown, B. (2010).** The Gifts of Imperfection: Letting Go of Who You Think You're Supposed to Be and Embracing

6

Embracing the Unknown: Resilience in the Face of Challenges

1. The Resilience Mindset: Dancing with Life's Storms

Ahoy, resilient voyager! Life is a magnificent dance, filled with twists and turns, dips and spins. In this section, we'll be your spirited dance partners, guiding you through the steps of embracing the unknown and cultivating resilience. So, slip on your dancing shoes, and let's boogie!

1. **Embracing Change:** Imagine yourself on a lively dance floor, the music pumping through your veins, and your body moving in sync with the rhythm. Life, too, is a dance of constant change. Embrace it with open arms, for change brings growth, new opportunities, and unexpected adventures. Step out of your comfort zone, dear dancer, and twirl through the ever-evolving choreography of life.

2. **Flexibility and Adaptability:** Like a skilled dancer who effortlessly adjusts to different rhythms, be flexible in the face of challenges. Bend, sway, and flow with the currents of life, knowing that your ability to adapt will keep you in harmony with the dance. Release attachments to rigid plans and expectations, allowing space for improvisation and creative solutions. Remember, dear improviser, that resilience lies in your ability to adapt.

3. **Building Inner Strength:** Close your eyes and feel the beat of your heart—the steady rhythm of your inner strength. Cultivate resilience by nurturing your physical, mental, and emotional well-being. Engage in activities that replenish your energy, such as exercise, meditation,

or spending time in nature. Strengthen your mind through positive affirmations, self-compassion, and cultivating a growth mindset. Your inner strength is the anchor that keeps you steady in turbulent waters.

4. **Seeking Support:** In the dance of life, you are never alone. Reach out your hand and let others join you on the dance floor. Seek support from loved ones, friends, or professionals who can provide guidance and a listening ear. Share your challenges, fears, and victories, knowing that vulnerability is a sign of strength. Together, you can create a dance of collective resilience.

5. **Finding Meaning in Adversity:** Just as a skilled dancer infuses every movement with intention, find meaning in the face of adversity. Seek the lessons and growth opportunities hidden within challenges. Reflect on the strength you've gained, the wisdom you've acquired, and the resilience you've cultivated. Every stumble is a chance to rise and dance even more beautifully.

6. **Cultivating Optimism:** Like a burst of confetti, optimism adds color and joy to your dance. Embrace a positive outlook, focusing on possibilities and opportunities. Challenge negative thoughts and reframe them with optimism and gratitude. Surround yourself with uplifting influences, inspiring stories, and laughter that lights up the dance floor. Remember, dear optimist, that resilience and joy are intertwined.

7. **Embracing Self-Compassion:** Imagine a warm embrace, wrapping you in love and acceptance. Extend that embrace to yourself, dear dancer. Embrace self-compassion as the gentle touch that soothes your soul during difficult times. Be kind and understanding toward yourself, acknowledging that mistakes and setbacks are part of the dance. Treat yourself with the same compassion you would extend to a dear friend who stumbled on the dance floor.

As you navigate the dance of life, remember that resilience is not about avoiding challenges but about embracing them with grace and fortitude.

With each step, you become more resilient, more attuned to the rhythm of the unknown. So, dance on, dear resilient soul, and let the beauty of your spirit shine through every twirl and sway.

References:

45. **Masten, A. S. (2001).** Ordinary magic: Resilience processes in development. American Psychologist, 56(3), 227-238.

46. **Fredrickson, B. L., Tugade, M. M., Waugh, C. E., & Larkin, G. R. (2003).** What good are positive emotions in crises? A prospective study of resilience and emotions following the terrorist attacks on the United States on September 11th, 2001. Journal of Personality and Social Psychology, 84(2), 365-376.

47. **Seligman, M. E. (2002).** Authentic happiness: Using the new positive psychology to realize your potential for lasting fulfillment. Free Press.

48. **Neff, K. D. (2003).** Self-compassion: An alternative conceptualization of a healthy attitude toward oneself. Self and Identity, 2(2), 85-101.

2. Bouncing Back: The Dance of Resilience

Greetings, tenacious dancer! In this section, we'll delve into the art of bouncing back, turning setbacks into comebacks, and transforming challenges into opportunities. Get ready to groove with resilience as we explore the dance floor of life!

1. **Acceptance and Emotional Agility:** Imagine yourself flowing through a dynamic dance routine, effortlessly adapting to each movement. Similarly, resilience requires embracing the full range of emotions that accompany challenges. Allow yourself to feel the sadness, frustration, or anger that may arise, knowing that emotions are an integral part of the dance. Practice emotional agility—acknowledge and accept your feelings, but don't let them define you. Embrace the power of choice, shifting your focus towards constructive actions.

2. **Cultivating Problem-Solving Skills:** Resilience is like a masterful improvisation—a dance move created on the spot. Develop your problem-solving skills to navigate obstacles with finesse. Break down challenges into manageable steps, brainstorm creative solutions, and seek different perspectives. Embrace a flexible and open-minded approach, knowing that there are often multiple paths to success. With each problem you solve, you become a more skilled dancer of resilience.

3. **Learning from Setbacks:** In the dance of resilience, setbacks are not stumbling blocks but valuable lessons. Embrace failure as an opportunity for growth and self-discovery. Reflect on the lessons learned, the skills honed, and the inner strength gained. Embrace the power of a growth mindset, where setbacks are seen as stepping stones toward success. With each setback, you grow wiser, more resilient, and better prepared for the next dance.

4. **Cultivating Self-Efficacy:** Picture a dancer radiating confidence, owning the stage with every step. Cultivate self-efficacy—the belief in your ability to overcome challenges. Celebrate past successes and

acknowledge your strengths and skills. Focus on building competence in areas relevant to your goals, seeking knowledge, training, and practice. With each achievement, your confidence soars, and resilience becomes second nature.

5. **Cultivating Optimism and Gratitude:** Like vibrant spotlights illuminating the dance floor, optimism and gratitude bring a sparkle to resilience. Embrace the power of positive thinking, focusing on possibilities, and maintaining hope even in the face of adversity. Practice gratitude, acknowledging the blessings and support in your life. Surround yourself with positivity, inspiring role models, and uplifting stories that ignite your spirit. Remember, dear optimist, that a positive mindset fuels resilience.

6. **Nurturing Self-Care:** Just as a dancer nourishes their body and mind, prioritize self-care in your resilience routine. Engage in activities that recharge your energy, whether it's practicing mindfulness, engaging in hobbies, or spending time in nature. Prioritize rest, nourishing foods, and regular exercise to support your well-being. Remember, dear dancer, that caring for yourself is not selfish but a necessary foundation for resilience.

7. **Cultivating Social Support:** In the dance of resilience, you are never alone on the floor. Surround yourself with a supportive network of friends, family, mentors, and communities. Seek connection, share your challenges, and ask for help when needed. Draw strength from the collective energy of those who believe in you. Together, you create a powerful dance of resilience.

As you embrace the unknown and dance with resilience, remember that setbacks are mere interludes in the grand choreography of life. Each step, whether forward or backward, contributes to your growth and strength. So, keep dancing, dear resilient soul, and let the rhythm of resilience guide you to new heights.

3. The Dance of Self-Compassion: Embracing Your Inner Light

Hey there, compassionate dancer! In this section, we'll explore the transformative power of self-compassion in the dance of resilience. Prepare to nurture yourself with kindness, embrace your inner light, and twirl through the dance floor of life with grace.

1. **Embracing Imperfection:** Picture a dancer on stage, flawlessly executing a routine. But here's a secret: even the most accomplished dancers make mistakes and stumble from time to time. Embrace your imperfections, dear dancer, for they make you beautifully human. Release the need for perfection and dance with self-compassion, accepting yourself exactly as you are. Remember, imperfections are the unique brushstrokes that paint the masterpiece of your resilience.

2. **Cultivating Self-Love:** Love is the music that fuels your dance of resilience. Shower yourself with self-love, dear dancer, celebrating your strengths, talents, and quirks. Treat yourself with the same tenderness and care you would extend to a cherished friend. Banish self-criticism and replace it with words of encouragement and affirmation. Let love be your guiding force, illuminating the path to resilience.

3. **Practicing Mindfulness:** In the midst of a lively dance, it's easy to get caught up in the whirlwind of thoughts and distractions. Practice mindfulness, bringing your awareness to the present moment. Tune in to the sensations in your body as you move, the rhythm of your breath, and the joy of each step. Embrace mindfulness as an anchor that keeps you grounded, allowing you to navigate challenges with clarity and compassion.

4. **Embracing Self-Forgiveness:** Just as partners in a dance forgive each other's missteps, forgive yourself for any perceived shortcomings or past mistakes. Release the weight of guilt or shame and embrace self-forgiveness. Understand that you are ever-evolving, learning, and

growing. Allow yourself the grace to let go of the past and move forward with compassion and renewed determination.

5. **Cultivating Resilient Self-Talk:** Imagine a chorus of supportive voices cheering you on as you dance. Cultivate resilient self-talk, replacing self-doubt and negativity with words of encouragement and empowerment. Challenge your inner critic and reframe self-limiting beliefs. Speak to yourself as your own best friend and ally. With each positive affirmation, you strengthen the foundation of your resilience.

6. **Connecting with Compassion:** Resilience is not a solo act—it thrives in connection and compassion. Extend kindness and empathy to others, nurturing the bonds that sustain your dance. Engage in acts of service, lend a listening ear, or offer a helping hand. In the dance of compassion, you create a ripple effect, inspiring others to embrace their own resilience.

7. **Cultivating Joy and Playfulness:** As you dance with resilience, don't forget to infuse joy and playfulness into your steps. Celebrate small victories, find moments of laughter, and savor the sheer delight of movement. Embrace the childlike spirit within you, allowing it to fuel your resilience. Remember, dear playful dancer, that joy is a powerful source of strength.

In the dance of resilience, self-compassion is the gentle touch that heals and nourishes your spirit. Embrace your uniqueness, love yourself unconditionally, and dance with grace and compassion. The world is your stage, and resilience is your dance of a lifetime.

References:

49. **Neff, K. D. (2011).** Self-compassion: Stop beating yourself up and leave insecurity behind. HarperCollins.

50. **Germer, C. K. (2009).** The mindful path to self-compassion: Freeing yourself from destructive thoughts and emotions. Guilford Press.

51. **Gilbert, P. (2009).** The compassionate mind: A new approach to life's challenges. New Harbinger

Publications.

This document is ©2023 Matti Charlton. Please contact me if you wish to do anything with it at retromatti [at] gmail [dot] com.